Anxiety Relief: How to conquer stress, fear, phobias, and panic attacks

I0477064

Table of Contents

How to Handle Panic Attacks

What it is Like to Have an Anxiety Attack

Overcoming your social anxiety disorder without medication

Forward

Anxiety disorders have become more prevalent and rampant today as it continues to affect more people. One contributing factor to anxiety disorders is stress at work as people struggle to take on several jobs to make ends meet. Other contributing factors are upbringing, family history, health issues, etc. People who suffer different kinds of anxiety disorders have varied symptoms to deal with. One thing that is unique with all types of anxieties and phobias is that they hold you back. The fact that they hold you back and try to stop you from reaching your goals and maximizing your potentials is the more reason why this is book is meant for you. One way to ensure you don't get stuck in the web on anxieties and fears that stop you from reaching for the moon in your chosen field is by following the techniques outlined in this book. Anxiety disorders can be mild, they can also be chronic. Following the wrong treatment techniques in an attempt to get rid of your phobias, fears and panic attacks will only result in making the problem more difficult to deal with. Most people who find themselves with anxiety disorders such as stage fright make the mistake of believing they can help their situation by taking some hard drugs or gulping some cups of rum before they mount the stage. Inasmuch as this might provide some immediate and short-term relief, it does not solve the problem in the long run. If there is anything alcohol and drugs do to your social anxiety disorders, it is making your condition worse and making your case appear more hopeless. Others believe they can beat their fears by avoiding situations that trigger their panic attacks. Avoiding the problem is never going to solve it-the best way to deal with your fears and phobias is to acknowledge them and the limits they have set before you and then defy those limits. Adopting the avoidance technique has never yielded any positive results. People who adopt the avoidance technique in college to skip discussion classes and debates end up performing below average in school. When they get a job, they still end up avoiding positions and posts that put them on the spotlight thereby hindering their own growths. These fears and phobias can be so overwhelming and powerful that one might be tempted to give up on life and everything worth believing in.

Introduction

Most people find themselves feeling anxious once in a while. However, anxiety can become a real issue once it starts interfering with your daily activities. Anxiety is one of the major symptoms of all anxiety disorders some of which are discussed below. But the good news is that anxiety can be treated easily using natural procedures, treatments and medication.

What exactly is anxiety?

It is natural for you to feel fearful or tense whenever you are anxious. You can equally have one or two unpleasant physical symptoms. For instance, you may find yourself dealing with issues like palpitations, fast heart rate, tremors, sweating, chest pain, headaches, dry mouth, fast breathing.

Part of the physical symptoms are caused by the brain which sends lots of messages down the nerves to different parts of the body whenever you are anxious. The nerve messages tend to make the lungs, heart and other body parts work very fast. Additionally, your body releases stress hormones like adrenaline into your bloodstream whenever you are anxious. These can equally act on muscles, heart and other parts of the body to cause some symptoms.

Anxiety is seen as normal during stressful situations, and can even be very helpful. For instance, most people will become anxious whenever they are threatened by a very aggressive person, or before a crucial race. The surge of nerve impulses and adrenaline which we often experience in response to very stressful situations can encourage a flight or fight response.

Anxiety is quite abnormal if you notice any of the following:

- Is out of proportion to the stressful situation; or

- Persists even after the stressful situation is no longer there, or the stress is minor; or

- Appears for no real reason when there is no stressful situation.

What exactly are Anxiety Disorders

There are several known conditions where anxiety is one of the major symptoms. If anxiety symptoms interfere with your normal day-to-day activities, it shows you may have developed some kind of anxiety disorder. You may also have anxiety disorder if you always find yourself worrying about developing anxiety symptoms. According to studies, one out of every 20 people suffer from one type of anxiety disorder or the day at one point in time. In some people, you can find some features of more than one type of anxiety disorder.

Chapter One

Overview

The major causes of anxiety disorders

Though there are no known causes of anxiety disorders yet; but anxiety disorders, like every other type of mental sickness, are not due to character flaws, personal weaknesses, or a substandard upbringing. As most scientists keep producing results from their researches on these disorders, it is now clear that these problems are caused by a number of factors, such as environmental stress and changes in the brain.

Like every other brain disease, anxiety disorders may result from problems emanating from the performance of the brain circuits that are responsible for the regulation of fears and other emotions. Studies have shown that severe and very long-lasting stress can cause anxiety disorders. Some researchers have shown that people suffering certain types of anxiety disorders tend to experience some changes in the brain structure in charge of controlling memories linked with very strong emotions. Additionally, studies have equally shown that anxiety disorders can run in families, which shows they can be partly inherited from one or both parents, just like the risk for cancer of heart disease. However, certain environmental factors, such as trauma or very significant events may trigger an anxiety disorder in people with inherited susceptibility to developing the condition.

How Common are Anxiety Disorders

Millions of adult Americans are affected by anxiety disorders. Most anxiety disorders start in childhood, adolescence, and early adulthood. They are more rampant in women than in men, and occur with the same frequency in African-Americans, whites, and Hispanics.

How to diagnose anxiety disorder

If there are symptoms of anxiety disorder, the doctor will start the evaluation by asking you about your medical history and carrying out physical examination. Though there are no specific lab tests to diagnose anxiety disorders, the doctor may adopt different tests to find out the physical illness responsible for the symptoms.

If there is no physical illness, you may have to be referred to a psychiatrist, psychologist, or another mental health expert who is trained to diagnose and treat mental illnesses. Psychologists and psychiatrists make use of specially designed assessment tools and interview to evaluate an individual for signs of anxiety disorders.

The bases for the diagnosis is always on the duration and intensity of the symptoms as reported by the patient. Problems with daily functioning brought about by the symptoms coupled with the doctor's observation of the attitude of the patient are equally taken into consideration. Based on the degree of dysfunction and symptoms, the doctor then decides if a specific anxiety disorder is involved.

How to treat anxiety disorders

Treating people with mental illnesses like mental disorders has become easier in the last two decades. Though the particular treatment approach to be adopted depends on the type of anxiety disorder involved, using one or a combination of some of the following therapies can provide you with the much needed relief for all types of anxieties.

- **Medication**

Drugs that have been found to be quite effective when it comes to reducing anxiety disorders include anxiety-reducing and anti-depressant drugs.

- **Psychotherapy**

Psychotherapy is a type of counseling that addresses all emotional responses to mental illness. It involves trained mental health experts talking to a person suffering anxiety disorder to help him or her understand the condition and how best to deal with it.

- **Cognitive behavioral therapy**

This is one type of psychotherapy in which the individual affected learns to master and change all thought patterns and behaviors that lead to unpleasant feelings. Other methods of treatment include:

- **Dietary and lifestyle changes.**
- **Relaxation therapy.**

How to Prevent Anxiety Disorders

Anxiety disorders cannot really be prevented; however, there are a number of steps you can take to control or reduce the symptoms.

- Quit or minimize the consumption of all caffeinated products such as tea, coffee, energy drinks, chocolate, and tea.

- Ask your pharmacist or doctor before you take any over-the-counter drugs or herbal remedies.

- Many come with certain chemicals that can increase the symptoms of anxiety.

- If you start feeling anxious more often without any known cause, seek counseling and support.

Generalized anxiety disorder risk factors

Any of the following factors can increase your risk of developing anxiety disorder.

- **Personality**

A person with a timid and negative temperament or who avoids anything that appears dangerous may be at a higher risk of anxiety disorder than others are.

- **Genetics**

There are proofs that anxiety disorders may run in some families.

- **Being female**

The number of women diagnosed with generalized anxiety disorder are somewhat higher than in men. Having generalized anxiety disorder does much more than making you worry. It can also do the following:

- Reduce your ability to carry out tasks quickly and efficiently because you find it hard to concentrate.

- Take your time and focus from other activities

- Sap your energy

- Disrupt your sleep

 Generalized anxiety disorder can also worsen other physical and mental conditions, such as;

  - Depression (which mostly occurs with generalized anxiety disorder)

  - Trouble sleeping(insomnia)

  - Substance abuse

  - Digestive or bowel problems

- Headaches

- Heart-health issues

Chapter Two

Major Types of Anxiety Disorders

Below is an overview of some of the major anxiety disorders.

Reactions to Stress

Anxiety can be one of the major symptoms as a reaction to very stressful situations. There are three known major types of reaction disorders.

Acute reaction to stress

This is also referred to as acute stress reaction. Acute means the symptoms develop very fast, over few minutes or some hours, reacting to the very stressful condition. These acute reactions to stress mostly occur after some very unexpected life crisis such as a severe accident, family problem, bereavement, bad news, etc. Symptoms can sometimes occur before an examination, a very important race or a concert performance.

The symptoms often settle quickly, but they can also last for a number of days or weeks. Apart from anxiety, other major symptoms include irritability, low mood, emotional ups and downs, poor concentration, poor sleep, the desire to be left alone.

Adjustment reaction

This is very similar to acute reaction, but then symptoms of adjustment reaction develop days or weeks after a certain stressful situation, as a reaction or an adjustment to the problem. For instance, as a reaction to a house move or divorce. Symptoms are similar to acute reaction to stress but may include depression. The symptoms mostly improve after a week or more.

Post-traumatic stress disorder

Post-traumatic stress disorder may come after a very severe trauma such as a life-threatening accident or a serious assault. The symptoms last for a month or more. Anxiety is the only symptom that can come and go. The major symptoms of post-traumatic stress disorder are:

- Recurring thoughts, images, memories, dreams, or flashback of the trauma, which are often distressing.

- You will find yourself trying to avoid thoughts, feelings, conversations, people, places, activities or anything else that is capable of triggering thoughts or memories of the trauma.

- Felling emotionally detached from others and numb. You may not find it easy to have loving feelings.

- You will often have pessimistic outlook for the future. You may find yourself losing interest in activities you once enjoyed.

- You may experienced increased arousal which you never had before the trauma set in. This may include irritation, sleeping difficulty, difficulty in concentration, and increased vigilance.

Phobic Anxiety disorders

A phobia is defined as a very strong dread or fear of a particular thing or event. The fear is out of proportion to the stack reality of the situation. Coming very close or in contact with the much dreaded situation causes anxiety. Sometimes, even the thought of the situation leads to anxiety. Consequently, you will always avoid the feared situation, which can restrict your life or cause severe suffering.

Social anxiety disorder

Social anxiety disorder, which is also known as social phobia is undoubtedly the most common phobia in existence. With social anxiety disorder, you are always very conscious of how others may judge you or, what they may think of you. As a result of this situation, you will always fear meeting people, or doing any kind of presentation that requires you to be in front of other people, especially strangers. You will always fear that you may end up acting in a very embarrassing way, and that others will end up thinking you are stupid, foolish, inadequate, weak, crazy, etc. You will always try to avoid such situations that will bring you in front of a crowd as much as possible. If you can't be excused from such situations, you become very anxious and distressed throughout the duration of such feared situation.

- **Agoraphobia**

This is yet another common type of anxiety disorder. Most people think it is just the fear of public places and open places, but it is much more than that. If you develop agoraphobia, you tend to have a number of fears of different situations and places. For instance, you may have the fear of:

- Going into shops, crowded and public places.

- Travelling in trains, planes, or buses.

- Being in a restaurant, cinema, etc where there is no easily accessible exit.

- Being in a lift or a bridge.

But they all come from the same underlying fear, which is the fear of being in a place where help cannot come easily, or where you feel it may not be easy to escape to your own home. Whenever you find yourself in such feared places, you will be very distressed and anxious to get out before you are harmed. To escape this anxiety, most people with this condition often stay in their homes where they feel safe.

Other Major Phobias

There are several other phobias of specific things and situations. Some examples are:

- Fear or being trapped in confined spaces.

- Fear of certain animals.

- Fear of injections.

- Fear of vomiting.

- Fear of choking

- Fear of being alone,

and many more.

Other Anxiety Disorders

Panic disorder

Panic disorder simply means you get recurring panic attacks. A panic attack is a severe attack of fear or anxiety that which occurs quiet suddenly, mostly without any warning, and for no known reason. The major physical symptoms of a panic attack can be quite severe and can include symptoms like thumping of the heart, feeling short of breath, trembling, chest pains, numbness, feeling faint, or needles and pins. Each panic attack can last between 5-10 minutes, but they can come in waves that can last for about two hours.

Generalized anxiety disorder

If your case is generalized anxiety disorder, then you have a lot of anxiety (feeling worried, tense and fearful) on most days. The condition persists long-term. Most of the above listed physical symptoms of anxiety may come and go. Your anxiety tends to be about different stressful situations at work or home, mostly about very minor issues. Sometimes, you may not even know why you are anxious. Additionally, you may usually experience three or more of the following symptoms:

- Feeling restless, edgy, or tensed most of the time.

- Getting tired and worn out too easily.

- Difficulty concentrating and a regular blank mind.

- Being irritable very often.

- Muscle tension.

- Insomnia. Most times, it is difficulty in getting off to sleep, or difficulty in staying asleep.

Mixed anxiety and depressive disorder

Most people experience anxiety as a symptom of depression. Other symptoms of depression include feelings of sadness, low mood, sleep problems, irritability, poor concentration, poor appetite, decreased sex drive, guilt, loss of energy, aches, headaches, palpitations and pains. Treatment for this condition is mainly aimed at easing depression, and the anxiety symptoms get eased in the process.

Obsessive-Compulsive disorder

Obsessive-compulsive disorder comprises of compulsions, obsessions, or both.

- Obsessions are recurring urges, images, or urges that cause you either disgust or anxiety. Common obsessions are fears about contamination, dirt, disasters, germs, violence, etc.

- Compulsions are actions or thoughts that you feel you have to do or repeat. Usually, a compulsion is a response to ease the anxiety brought about by the obsession. A good example is a repeated washing of hands in response to the obsession about contacting germs through dirt. Other good examples of compulsion include checking, cleaning, touching, counting, and hoarding of objects.

What are the major or minor symptoms?

It is normal for you to get nervous or anxious from time to time, especially when treading unknown grounds. Situations such as speaking in public, or going through financial difficulties can get on your nerves. For a number of people, however, anxiety gets too frequent, or even forceful, that it begins to run their lives. How can you tell if your own anxiety issue has crossed the line between normal and disorder? Sometimes, it is hard to tell. Anxiety can come in different forms and patterns-such as phobia, panic attacks, social anxiety, etc, like we have earlier outlined and the distinction between a normal anxiety and an official diagnosis isn't always very clear. Once you start experiencing any of the symptoms listed below more regularly, then it is time to pay your doctor a visit.

Excessive worry

The peak of generalized anxiety disorder, which is known to be the broadest type of anxiety-is worrying rather too much about everyday issues, big and small. But when can we say the worry has become too much?

In the case of generalized anxiety disorder, it means having recurrent anxious thoughts on most days in the week, for about six months. Also, the anxiety must become so bad that it starts interfering with daily life and is accompanied by very noticeable symptoms, such as fatigue.

The clear distinction between having normal anxiety and anxiety disorder is whether your emotions are causing lots of dysfunctions and sufferings.

Sleep problems

Trouble falling asleep or staying asleep for long can be traced to a number of health-related issues, both psychological and physical. It is not very unusual to toss and turn with anticipation or uncertainty on the night before a job interview or a big speech.

But if you find yourself lying awake chronically, worried or agitated- about certain issues like money, or nothing in particular, it may be a clear sign you have anxiety disorder. By some reliable analysis, nearly half of people suffering from generalized anxiety disorder have sleep problems.

Another sign that shows you may be suffering from anxiety disorder is if you often wake up feeling a bit wired, with a racing heart, and you are not able to calm yourself down no matter how much you try.

Irrational fears

Some anxiety is far from generalized; on the contrary, it is often attached to a specific situation or thing-such as crowds, animals, or flying. If the fear becomes uncontrollable, out of proportion with the risk involved and a bit disruptive, it is a telltale sign of phobia, or a type of anxiety.

Although phobias can become quite crippling, they are not always obvious. In fact, they may not show up until such a time when you are confronted by a specific situation and discover you are not able to overcome your fears. For instance, if you are afraid of snakes, you can go for several years without having a single problem as a result of your phobia, but when your kid suddenly starts talking about going camping with his mates, you remember you need to take them to your doctor for medical checkup.

Muscle Tension

Near-constant muscle tension-whether it has to do with clenching your jaw, flexing your muscles throughout your body, or balling your feet-often accompanies some types of anxiety disorders. This symptom can be so pervasive and persistent that people who have endured it for years can stop noticing its existence after sometime.

Exercising regularly can go a long way to help keep your muscle tension under control, but the tension may resurface if an injury or other sudden events spring up to disrupt your workout schedules and habits. Suddenly you find yourself a wreck because you lack the willpower to handle your anxiety in that way which may result in restlessness and irritability.

Chronic indigestion

Anxiety often begins in the mind, but it often shows itself in the body through physical symptoms, such as chronic digestive problems. Irritable bowel syndrome, a condition characterized by cramping, bloating, constipation, stomachaches, and/or diarrhea, is basically a form of anxiety in the digestive tract.

Irritable bowel syndrome is not always related to some kind if anxiety, but they often accompany each other when they strike, and can make the effect of each other more unbearable. The gut is quite sensitive to psychological stress- and, vice versa, both the social and physical discomfort that come with chronic digestive problems can make a person with this problem experience more serious anxiety.

Stage fright

Most people are used to getting a few butterflies before addressing a group of people or when they are in the spotlight. But if the fear becomes so strong that no amount of practice or coaching will alleviate it, or if you spend much time worrying and thinking about it, you may develop some kind of social anxiety disorder.

People suffering from social anxiety disorder tend to worry for several days or weeks leading up a certain event or situation they cannot escape from. And when they manage to go through with such event or situation, they tend to become very uncomfortable and may dwell on it for a very long time afterwards, wondering how the audience judged their performance or presentation.

Self-consciousness

Social anxiety disorder does not always involve talking to a large crowd or being the center of attention. In most cases, the anxiety is provoked by daily situations like making-one-on-one conversation at a party, or eating and drinking in front of even the smallest crowd.

In these situations, people suffering social anxiety disorder feel like all eyes are watching them, and they often end up blushing, trembling, nauseated, sweating profusely, and incoherent speech. These symptoms can become so severe that it becomes hard for them to meet new people, maintain healthy relationships, and advance at work or in school.

Panic

Panic attacks can be quite terrifying: picture any sudden, gripping feeling of helplessness and fear that can last for a couple of minutes, accompanied by scary physical symptoms such as a pounding or racing heart, breathing problems, tingling or numb hands, weakness, sweating, chest pain, and a feeling of hotness or coldness.

Though not every panic attack is related to an anxiety disorder, but people who experience them often may be diagnosed with panic disorder. Panic with this condition live with the fears about how, when, why and where their next panic attack might happen, and they tend to avoid places where such attacks have occurred in the past.

Flashback

Reliving a very disturbing or traumatic event such as a sudden death of a loved one, a violent encounter is the hallmark of post-traumatic stress disorder, which is known to share certain features with anxiety disorders. Before post-traumatic stress disorder become recognized as a standalone condition, it was often seen as a type of anxiety disorder.

But flashbacks may also occur with other types of anxiety. According to some researches, such as the 2006 study in the *journal of anxiety disorders,* some people with social anxiety have post-traumatic stress disorders such as flashbacks of experiences that might not have seem obviously traumatic, like being ridiculed publicly. These people may even try to avoid anything that reminds them of the experience.

Perfectionism

The obsessive and finicky mind-set known as perfectionism accompanies anxiety disorders. If you are always judging yourself or you have a lot of anticipatory anxiety about making mistakes and performing below your standards, you probably have anxiety disorder.

Perfectionism is especially common in obsessive-compulsive disorder, which like post-traumatic disorder has always been seen as a type of anxiety disorder. Obsessive-compulsive disorder can happen subtly, a good example is someone who cannot leave home for two or three hours without the right makeup, and often starts all over to makeup before leaving the house.

Compulsive behaviors

In order to be diagnosed with obsessive-compulsive disorder, a person's intrusiveness and obsessiveness must come with compulsive behavior, whether it is mental like telling yourself "everything will be fine" repeatedly or physical like straightening items and hand-washing.

Obsessive thinking and compulsive behavior become full-blown disorder when the need to complete the behaviors-which is also referred

to as rituals starts driving your life.

Chapter Three

How to deal with your fears

Intention has been identified as a very important factor when it comes to dealing with fear. Scholars are of the opinion that intentions are related to fear because if you can learn to focus your mind on the potential positive outcomes of whatever situation you fear, you are likely to face less fear in most of such situation.

It is quite easy to allow fear play a part in your daily life. Life gives you several opportunities to face your fears, knowing how to deal with your fears and overcome them will save you from lots of difficulties in the long run. There are several key facts that can break down your fears and allow you focus on your goals.

Below are five important techniques that will help you overcome the fears life will shove your way in your daily life.

- **Start Small**

Fear comes in different sizes and shapes. Facing your fears does not have to be a very big gesture. Supposing your fear is related to meeting new people, you will always have difficulty starting a relationship. One way to take care of your fears is to break down your anxiety into smaller, more manageable challenges. Instead of worrying about how to meet the right person for you, you can focus more on how to make new friends. Focusing on smaller more manageable goals will help you worry less about the end results. No matter how big your fears might be, scaling them down to smaller challenges will be beneficial in the long run. The same technique still works if your fear is the fear of speaking in public. Engage small groups in discussions, accept to talk to small crowds, and that will help you gain more confidence to take on speaking to a large audience. Step out of your comfort zone slowly and start moving towards your goal.

- **Believe**

While it may not be easy for you to achieve your desired results immediately, it is important to hold on to the belief that in time, you will achieve the goals you have set to conquer your fears. Believing that achievement is not just possible, but probable will go a long way to soften your fears.

Take your mind back to one past event that had seemed terrible at that time, but for certain circumstances was allowed to happen and in the end it brought about a greater and more amazing event. That is a very good proof that the world is not against you, but rather working with you and in your favor.

- **Write it down**

One great way to work through our fears is to make a list of them. Writing in a journal can go a long way to help you overcome certain fears like the fear of rejection, not meeting the right person, not being up to standard, not having adequate knowledge on a particular issue, not having the courage to face a crowd, etc. Write about the experiences you had on dates you went to, events you attended, public functions you featured in, discussion classes you took part in and how each of them made you feel afterwards. This technique will help you chart your progress and help you keep a list of what you have learned in the past. Writing down your fears helps you accept that things are evolving, even when they seem not to, and this brings you to the next important technique for conquering fear: acceptance.

- **Accept whatever develops and what fails to develop**

One important thing you must do when dealing with your fears is to accept the fact that you have a serious fear issue. Face the facts and accept that your fears can destroy you if you don't destroy them. According to Dalai Lama, "If you have some fear of suffering or pain, you must make sure you examine whether you can do something about it. If you can do something about it, then you don't need to worry; if there is nothing you can do about your fears, then there is also no need to get yourself all worried and worked up".

- **Learn to Let go**

Letting go can be a great challenge to overcoming your fears. Most times, we cling to something because we believe it empowers us; however, holding on to things we ought to let go only weakens us. Once you accept what may or may not be changed easily, the next thing is to detach yourself from the outcome. Letting go of your fears allows you to focus on the present moment and not on the fear itself.

Chapter Four

Major Treatments for anxiety disorders and phobias

The major aim of most treatments for treating anxiety disorders and phobias is to help you reduce the symptoms so that the anxiety disorder and its attendant effects can no longer affect your everyday life. These treatments may include one or more of the following:

NON-Medication TREATMENTS

- **Understanding**

Understanding the cause of the symptoms, and talking things over with a friend, family member or health practitioner may help. In particular, most people worry that most physical symptoms of anxiety, such as palpitations, are due to a physical ailment. This can make the anxiety worse. Understanding the fact that you have a serious anxiety disorder is not enough to get you cured, but it will go a long way to help you on the journey to getting over the problem.

- **Counseling**

This may help some people with certain types of anxiety disorders. For instance, counseling which focuses on problem-solving skills may give some kind of help to people suffering generalized anxiety disorder.

Anxiety Management Courses

These maybe an option for certain conditions, if courses are offered in your area. The courses may include: problem-solving skills, learning how to relax, coping strategies, and group support.

Cognitive and behavioral therapy

The therapies, if available in your area, can work well for persisting anxiety disorders and phobias:

- Cognitive therapy is based on the notion that certain thought patterns can fuel, or trigger, certain mental health problems such as depression and anxiety. Your therapist helps you to understand your present thought patterns-most importantly, to identify any unhelpful, harmful, and false notions, beliefs, or thoughts you may have that can likely result in anxiety or depression.

- The major aim is then to change you thought pattern in order to avoid these ideas. Also, to help make your thought pattern more helpful and realistic. Therapy is mostly done in weekly sessions of about 50 minutes each, for a couple of weeks. You have to participate very actively, and get homework in-between sessions. For instance, you may be asked to make a diary of your thoughts which occur when you get anxious or develop some physical symptoms of anxiety.

- Behavioral therapy aims at changing any behaviors which are considered either unhelpful or harmful. For instance, with phobias your behaviors or response to feared object is harmful, and the therapist aims to help you change this. Various techniques are used, depending on the conditions and circumstances. Several sessions are also required for a course of therapy just like we saw in the cognitive therapy.

- Cognitive behavioral therapy is a blend of the two where you stand to benefit from changing both thoughts and behaviors. Both cognitive and behavioral therapies do not look into past events; rather, they aim at or try to change your present thought patterns and/or behaviors.

- **Self-help**

There are several national groups that offer quality information, support and advice. These groups, your doctor or a practicing nurse, may help connect you to some local groups for face-to-face support. You can equally get leaflets, books, tapes and videos on combating stress and relaxation. They teach very simple but effective deep-breathing techniques and several other measures to relieve stress, help you relax better, and possibly get rid of your anxiety symptoms.

Medication

Antidepressant medicines

These are commonly used for treating depression, but also help you reduce the symptoms of anxiety even when you are not depressed. They work by interfering with your brain chemicals known as the neurotransmitters such as serotonin which may be one of the causes of anxiety disorders.

- Antidepressants do not work immediately. It takes about 2-4 weeks before their effects can be felt and the anxiety symptoms begin to give way. One common problem is that most people stop the medication after one week or more because they feel it is not helping them at all. This is often too soon to measure the effect of the medication on the condition.

- Antidepressants are not really tranquilizers, and are not usually addictive.

- Several types of antidepressants exist, each comes with its various pros and cons. Most differ in their possible side-effects. However, selective serotonin reuptake inhibitor antidepressants are the most commonly used for anxiety disorders.

- **NB:** after some people with anxiety problems start taking some antidepressants, the symptoms of the anxiety disorder may get worse for some days before they start noticing some improvements. Your doctor or nurse may want to keep you under check in the first few weeks to know if you have any kind of problems.

Benzodiazepines

Benzodiazepines like diazepam was once the most commonly prescribed medication for anxiety. They were often regarded as the minor tranquilizers but they do come with some serious known side-effects. They are often very effective for easing symptoms of anxiety. The major problem is that they can be very addictive and can easily lose their effect on your anxiety symptoms if you keep taking them for over a few week. They can equally make you drowsy. They are no longer used much for persistent anxiety conditions and short-term, or once in awhile to help you get over some very bad spell if you suffer from persistent anxiety symptoms.

Buspirone

Buspirone is sometimes included in the prescription for the treatment of general anxiety disorder. Though it is not yet clear how this medicine works, it is known to be an active anti-depressant medicine. It is not addictive and is believed to affect the production and circulation of serotonin in the brain. Serotonin is suspected to be involved in causing anxiety symptoms.

Beta-blocker medicines

A beta-blocker such as propranolol, can help ease some of these physical symptoms like trembling, heart thumping, etc. They may not have a direct effect of the mental symptoms like worry.

However, some people find it easier to relax if their physical symptoms are eased. This works better in short-lived severe anxiety disorder. For instance, if you get more anxious before you begin your performance in a concert then a beta-blocker may help you ease the tension and anxiety.

In some cases, a combination of treatments like antidepressants and cognitive therapy may work better than using only one of the treatments.

Alcohol and anxiety.

Though alcohol has been found to ease the symptoms for a short period, don't make the mistake of believing you can cure your anxiety by drinking alcohol. In the long run, drinking alcohol cannot cure anxiety disorders. Drinking alcohol often to calm jumbled nerves can result in problem drinking and may make the anxiety and depression problems worse in the long run. If you are taking alcohol or some street drugs to ease anxiety, you need to see a doctor as soon as possible before things get worse.

Chapter Five

How to Deal With Generalized Anxiety Disorder

15 TIPS FOR GENERALIZED ANXIETY DISORDER

Anxiety alert-Why you should know

Technically put, anxiety is nothing but apprehension over an upcoming event. We sometimes anticipate the future with very scary predictions that may not have any kind of basis in truth and reality. In our daily lives, the common physical and emotional symptoms of anxiety may include increased heart rate, poor concentration in school and work, sleeping problems, and just being an anxious wreck to everyone around including family, friends and colleagues.

Stress and anxiety are often physical and emotional responses to perceived dangers that may not be real most of the time. Since most of us don't face situations where we need to run from some wild and ferocious tigers and the likes, most of the dangers we face come from little issues such as an overfilled email inbox, losing our keys before we run out the door, morning rush hour, etc. Luckily, it is quite easy to overcome this kind of stress with very little changes added to our lifestyles throughout the day.

However, if you feel you have very severe case of anxiety disorder, you may need to speak to your doctor to get professional help and advice. There are several options available to you when it comes to managing your anxiety disorder and its attendant symptoms. But if what you need are ways to minimize your daily anxiety, below are the most helpful tips you can find on this issue to help you get back to your collected and calm state.

- **Get adequate sleep**

Inconsistent sleep can have some very dire consequences. It does not stop at affecting our physical health, but lack of sleep can contribute to your overall stress and anxiety levels. It sometimes turn into a very vicious cycle, since anxiety mostly leads to serious disruptions in sleep. Whenever you are beginning to feel very anxious, sleep for seven to nine hours and observe what a few days of adequate sleep can do to your stress and anxiety levels throughout the day.

- **Smile**

When work keeps you busy all day, it is advisable you take some break to get on some refreshing giggles. According to studies, laughter can reduce the major symptoms of anxiety and depression quite significantly. You can find something funny to read or watch to help you calm your nerves.

- **De-clutter your brain**

It can be either physical or mental clutter or both. A very messy workspace can make relaxation more difficult and make it seem like you work is never going to end. Some always take about 15 minutes to tidy things up at home and work, and form the habit of keeping things clean and as anxiety-free as possible. This will go a long way to help you think rationally and there won't be much room for anxiety.

- **Express gratitude**

Studies have shown that expressing gratitude helps you reduce your anxiety levels, especially when you get enough rest. You can begin a gratitude journal to get in the mindset of appreciation, and out of an overwhelmed mindset.

- **Eat Right**

Anxiety can sometimes throw your body out of order: Your appetite might change, or you may start craving certain foods. But to give the body the much needed support, eat foods that contain more of vitamin B and Omega-3, as well as some wholegrain carbohydrates. Studies have shown vitamin B to be essential for mental health, and omega-3 useful for reducing the symptoms of anxiety and depression. Wholegrain carbs are effective for the regulation of serotonin levels, the neurotransmitter that helps us feel good and remain calm. Though your cravings might not want to agree, but studies have shown that eating processed and sugary foods can increase the symptoms of anxiety.

- **Practice breathing**

Breathing can help determine your stress and anxiety levels all through the day and help prevent panic attacks. Very short and shallow breaths signify anxiety and stress levels in your brain and body. On the other hand, breathing consciously, plus strengthening and lengthening the breath sends positive signals to the brain that everything is ok.

- **Meditate**

We have always been told that engaging in meditations can help you relax your brains and muscles, but more recent studies have shown that it equally helps to increase the number of grey matter in the brain. This is very essential in rewiring the brain for less stress. Different recent studies have shown the positive effects meditation has on stress, anxiety, and mood. Meditation is also a very effective way of observing the brain, which lets us understand how our mind produces anxiety-provoking thoughts. Understanding the brain's patterns can help you create a healthy distance from such thoughts.

- **Create the Vision board**

If thinking about the future gives you a scary feeling, try changing your thoughts about what lies ahead. Most times, the mere practice of setting attainable goals can remove the anxiety about future unknowns. Take about an hour to formulate a vision board that helps you create excitement about possibilities and projects to come. You can create an e-vision using pinterest to get some pinspirations. You can make use of the T.H.I.N.K tool while making creating this vision board. Ask yourself if your thoughts are True, Helpful, Inspirational, Necessary, and Kind. If they are not, dump them.

- **Play Around**

Kids and animals seem to be born with an innate ability to play, without any stressful thoughts about their overfilled inboxes. You will have to take responsibility of your own playtime until business offices start giving recess breaks. You can get out of your head by offering to babysit for an afternoon or to take a friends dog for a walk.

- **Be silent**

Plan for a time when you can disconnect yourself from everything and everyone. Begin with durations that are both doable and sustainable for you, even if it is just for five minutes. That means no phone calls, no emails, no news, no TV, nothing. Let everyone know they will not be able to reach you within these few worry-free   minutes. There are some evidence that too much noise can increase your stress levels, so schedule some sacred silent time among all the commotion of your daily life.

- **Worry**

Yes, you can cause yourself to freak out, but only for some short period of time. When you have a heavy load on your mind about an issue, or you feel most certain something terrible is about to happen, commit to creating that worry for about 20 minutes and not more. Think of every possible outcome of the scenario and think about a feasible game plan, and then stop thinking about it once the time has elapsed. Involve a friend to in immediately the allotted the allotted has gone by to keep you away from exceeding the time limit. Or schedule some of the playtime immediately after that period.

- **Plan ahead**

Fight anxious thoughts ahead of time by making preparations for the day ahead. Try making some schedule or to-do-list and develop some habits that can help you increase productivity. So instead of spending about 15 minutes every morning frantically searching for your keys, form the habit of keeping the in the same place the moment you get home every day. Lay your cloths out the night before, pack your gym bag and place it close to the exit door, or prepare lunch ahead of time. Pay attention to how you can remove the anxiety-producing beliefs from your head by prepping before they start popping up.

- **Visualize anything positive**

Whenever you are confronted with very anxious thoughts, take some minutes to visualize yourself taking care of the situation with ease, calm, and clarity. Remove your attention from the present mental state; just focus on the feeling of smooth-sailing through the storm.

This technique is known as guided imagery or guided visualization and can help reduce signs of stress.

- **Smell a relaxing aroma**

Sniff some oils with very calming effects. Basil, chamomile, and anise are some great choices you could make. These oils reduce your body tension and help increase your mental clarity.

- **Hang out**

People with social support react less negatively to stress than those who live solo. This maybe because socializing has been found to stimulate the production of the hormone oxytocin, which has some anxiety-reducing effects. So next time you notice a freak-out creeping in, grab some friends and go for a walk or engage in a group chat.

5 More Tips for Controlling Generalized Anxiety Disorder

Generalized Anxiety Disorder is a situation that makes you feel anxious and tense almost all the time over issues that wouldn't have bothered you normally. Feeling tense and anxious most of the time will take the very meaning and excitement out of your life.

Why do you feel anxious and tense most times?

There are several issues that can make you worried and tense most times, some of these issues can be financial worries, relationship problems, bad bosses, unresolved traumas, bad diet, fear of not fulfilling expectations adequately, as well as excessive stimulant consumption.

Once you are diagnosed with generalized anxiety disorder, you need to try the following listed techniques.

Remember it is not abnormal

Always remind yourself that all the symptoms of generalized anxiety disorder you have been feeling are all part of the feelings we are supposed to get once in a while normally. Don't be scared by the clinical and psychiatric diagnoses. Even when you feel like a pack of wolves are on your trail, it can be as a result of a build-up of stress.

Pay attention to what gives you stress and try to reduce it.

Lots of problems can crop up at the same time to give you a very high intimidating pack of stresses. Try to find out when the generalized anxiety disorder began. Find out what was going on in your life as at when it started. Were you experiencing an abnormally higher stress levels than usual? Even a few nights of inadequate sleep can be enough to stir up intense anxiety in people.

Never forget you are quite safe.

The high level of trepidation, anxiety, and foreboding often noticed in people with Generalized Anxiety Disorder is normal, even helpful, in continuous physical unsafe circumstances. If you feel physically unsafe at the moment, then you must take the necessary steps immediately to make sure you are safe. Most times, the things we worry about don't really exist or they are not as bad as we take them to be.

Don't worry about worry

One very commonly reported symptom of Generalized Anxiety Disorder is the worry about things that should not have been worried about. This happens due to the fact that your body always seeks to justify your emotions when you have strong feelings. In this kind of situation, your body seems to try creating a container for your feelings. A good example is when you have been seething with intense anger over a certain issue, you can go out in the street still angry and find yourself angry about non-issues like a little old woman who keeps talking right in front of you while you are on a queue, the strange and unconventional way most strangers look, the way people are talking, and several other such scenario. This will continue until you are able to calm yourself down. Generalized Anxiety Disorder makes you search for things you can be worried about. Always remember this to enable you put worries where they belong and look at them the way they should be seen.

The Takeaway

In the ideal world, we wouldn't consciously come up with thoughts that result in stress and anxiety. But because we are humans, worrying is inevitable, especially when we have things to worry about. So whenever we do start to freak, there are several little steps we can take to change our thought patterns, calm our brains, relax our bodies, and get ourselves back into the game. And, as usual, make sure you check with a qualified psychotherapist if these tips and advice contained in this book do not produce the required results you will need more professional help to tackle more serious anxiety problems.

Chapter Six

Things that can trigger anxiety disorder

Everyone gets restless, frazzled, and anxious-but once you start experiencing constant anxiety and can't trace it to anything, you could have anxiety disorder. Doctors make diagnosis of generalized anxiety disorder when patients have anxiety symptoms like difficulty concentrating , frequent headaches, and constant worry for over six months without any good reason. Though the causes of anxiety disorders are not known yet, but certain triggers of anxiety disorders have been identified such as thyroid problems and weight-loss supplements.

Heart Problems

If you have ever had a panic attack, it means you are quite familiar with how your hands can get moist, you can't catch your breath-and your heart feels like it will pound right out of your chest. But most anxieties can be caused by problems with your heart. Most people after they have gone through some heart-surgeries and heart attack experience some anxiety symptoms such as shortness of breath and palpitation. These symptoms can last up to a year or more, and mostly occur in women.

- **Alcohol and drugs**

People with anxiety disorders, especially social anxiety disorders are about three times more likely to have issues with drugs and alcohol. But that is not all: Alcohol and drugs abuse can equally lead to anxiety disorder and an anxiety attack. People suffering social anxiety who abuse alcohol have been found to have serious anxiety symptoms-as well as several other emotional problems and health conditions. No matter what problem comes first, a combination of alcohol, drugs, and anxiety can form a very vicious cycle.

- **Caffeine**

Caffeine is a very powerful stimulant and can be a very bad thing for someone suffering anxiety disorder. In fact, the effect of caffeine on your body can be likened to a very frightening event. This is because caffeine stimulates your fight or fright response, and researches have shown that this can worsen your anxiety attacks. And just like the known symptoms of anxiety, the intake of several cups of coffee can leave you feeling moody, nervous, and awake all through the night.

- **Medications**

Certain medications come with very ugly side effects-they can cause severe anxiety symptoms or even trigger an anxiety attack. Prescriptions to be careful with include asthma drugs, thyroid drugs, over the counter decongestants and combination cold remedies can put at risk. And if you suddenly stop taking drugs to control your anxiety symptoms, the sudden withdrawal can cause anxiety symptoms.

Weight Loss Supplements

Most over-the-counter weight loss supplements come with anxiety-producing side effects. Saint

John's wort side effects may include insomnia, and green tea extracts (which claim to suppress appetite) contain lots of caffeine.

Your Thyroid Gland

Your thyroid gland is a butterfly-shaped gland in the front of your neck that produces thyroid hormones. This hormone is very important for the regulation of your metabolism and energy levels. But if your thyroid produces lots of hormones, it can lead to anxiety symptoms, such as irritability, heart palpitations, nervousness, and sleeplessness. If you notice anxiety symptoms coupled with weight loss, swelling in the neck, fatigue, heat intolerance, or weakness, you need to have your thyroid gland checked by your doctor.

Stress

Stress and anxiety are known to go hand in hand. Stress is known to result in serious anxiety symptoms, and anxiety can worsen the stress. When you are very tense, you may equally resort to other behaviors that make anxiety worse such as drug abuse, smoking, or alcohol abuse. Don't forget that anxiety and stress are often accompanied by physical symptoms such as headache, stomachache, dizziness, dry mouth, and sweating. If you have symptoms of anxiety whose origin cannot be traced, you need to talk to your doctor. It is important to note that all anxiety disorders are quite treatable.

Chapter Seven

How to Handle Panic Attacks

It may not be easy to avoid your anxiety during a panic attack, but learning the right techniques to adopt can help you get your anxiety back under control.

Panic attacks can be quite terrifying when they strike. These attacks can stem from profound anxiety that can cause intense palpitations and make your knees weak. Panic attacks can make it hard for you to catch your breath, they can also cause you chest pain and dizziness. Sometimes when under panic attacks, you may think you are having a heart attack. A panic attack lasts only for a few minutes, but it can leave you frightened and uneasy.

What causes panic attacks

A panic attack and its symptoms of great anxiety can come so unexpectedly, out of the blue. While the panic attack itself may be quite brief and short-lived, it can leave a long-lasting fear of having another attack in its wake. When these panic attacks and the fear of having other attacks come too often, the individual is said to be suffering panic disorder, a serious type of anxiety disorder. People suffering panic attacks always worry about having such attacks, and may end up avoiding all situations that make them remember the previous attack. In the long run, people suffering panic disorder discover they are not really afraid of the particular situation they have been avoiding, but rather experiencing more panic attacks. Fortunately, you can live without having these fears of a possible panic attack. There are certain strategies you can adopt to help you take control of your physical symptoms and manage your anxiety as well.

How to Take Control of Your Panic Attacks

The best way to avoid future panic attacks is by learning to control your anxiety so that once you start noticing the symptoms of panic attack, you can keep your mind and body calm till the symptoms go away. People who experience these panic attacks have to learn how best to manage their feelings of panic. Though medication can be quite effective, cognitive-behavioral therapy remains one of the best techniques for managing anxiety and panic disorders. People with panic disorder have to be aware that their thoughts are capable of triggering a physical reaction, which often results in a panic attack.

To gain control over your panic disorder, it is very important you learn and practice relevant anxiety management techniques. Strategies that you can use to help you curtail a panic attack include:

- **Breathing slowly and deeply**

Anxiety can make you breathe very quickly, which makes all the symptoms of a panic attack, both physical and mental worse. When you start feeling panicky, make sure you take some slow, deep breaths to calm your mind and body.

- **Stop and think**

Whenever your thoughts start spinning out of control, simply instruct yourself to stop. Organize yourself and decide what it will require to bring your mind to its normal calm state.

- **Think Positively**

Remove all negative thoughts from your mind, and remind yourself you are in charge here. Think about past situations when you have been able to manage such anxious situations quite successfully without fuss.

- **Stand up for yourself**

If you need to leave a particular venue or situation, do so or inform someone you need to leave. Don't be shy to ask for help. Becoming upset will not help the situation and will end up getting you more upset. So take a walk and blow off some steam if that is what you need to calm yourself down.

- **Relax your muscles**

One of the physical effects of anxiety is that it causes your entire body to tense up, so make some efforts to calm your muscles, from your toes to your face.

You don't have to wait for the panic attack to strike before you start practicing these techniques, It is important to engage in regular practice of these techniques and learn o manage your anxiety gradually. When you become more confident that you can handle your panic attacks better, you can easily walk out the door each day with calmer breaths.

What it is Like to Have an Anxiety Attack

Sweating, flushing, pounding heart rate, sore chest: You might mistake these sensations as signs of a heart attack, but it could be nothing other than a panic attack.

I once heard of a Los Angeles entrepreneur Neal Sideman was in the middle of his regular workout at the gym when he started feeling lighthearted and noticed his heart was pounding uncontrollably. He became alarmed about his heart-he never suspected a panic attack.

However, a visit to his doctor the next day and an EKG proved his heart was in perfect condition. According to his doctor, what he experienced was just some symptoms of anxiety.

Signs of Anxiety and Panic Attacks

An anxiety and panic attack comes on too suddenly, with its symptoms lasting only a few minutes. Before doctors can diagnose a panic attack, they lookout for at least four of the following signs: trembling, sweating, choking sensation, shortness of breath, nausea, vomiting, chest pain, dizziness, fear of death, fear of losing your mind, feelings that there are dangers lurking around, heart palpitations, flushing, and feeling a very intense need to escape.

Stress, Anxiety, and Panic:

Gideon's story

In the words of Gideon my friend and colleague, his attack occurred in the early 90s, and most people seriously believed he could have repeated panic attacks in the future. So, he got home and shared the story of his panic attack with his family hoping all would be fine, not knowing that another attack was about to hit in a week's time.

Several years after that experience, he can now tell the story of his panic attacks more clearly. According to him, the stress at his work place where we worked 16 hours a day on the average did him a lot of harm. He had a sick and dying friend, and above all, he was involved in super heavy workout regimen at the gym near his house with his trainer. So he had a combination of physical, emotional, and a whole lot of financial stresses. According to Gideon, there were visible signs of anxiety in his childhood and teen years as well as in other members of his family.

At that moment when he was undergoing the panic attack, he didn't know exactly what to think about because you cannot possibly know what a panic attack is until you have gone through one. His second panic attack was more severe than the first one and can be termed a full-blown panic attack. According to him, he thought he was going to die as a result of that second panic attack. The thought of an imminent death was not the only thought on his mind. He thought he would die, pass out, go crazy, or have a heart attack.

He recalled how terrified he was during the first and second attacks, and the response he decided to adopt happened to be one response that can really worsen the situation of a panic attack. His response was to avoid situations that reminded him of when and where he had those attacks. He thought he could just get smart, take care of himself, and not go out much. He found ways to build his business without having to leave his home or office. After his first panic attack on a freeway, he decided to avoid driving on freeways-a very tough decision to take in a city like Los Angeles. He kept avoiding all activities that could lead to panic attacks, but that never provided the much needed solution for his panic disorder. After about three years, he suddenly realized his panic attacks were getting worse despite all his efforts to curb them.

How to Cope With Anxiety and Panic Attacks

Desperate for urgent help, he got in touch with the Anxiety and Depression Association of

America, which made a list of all experienced therapists on panic attacks and anxiety disorders available to him. This was how he began his journey towards overcoming panic attacks. He found a certified therapist who understood what panic disorder was quite well, understood agoraphobia, and knew cognitive behavioral therapy. He was also introduced into meditation as a part of his treatment regimen.

Cognitive behavioral therapy has been found to help people suffering panic disorder and agoraphobia reduce their symptoms for a reasonable period of time, like two years.

According to experts in the field of panic disorder, people suffering anxiety disorder can always get help if they can seek professional help after the first one or two panic attacks. When you go for professional help, your doctor or therapist will want to know the symptoms you have been getting, the situations when such symptoms occur and might recommend some additional medical testing to rule out the possibility of other health issues.

Make sure you don't wait too long before you seek the help of a professional because that might result in more difficulties in trying to unlearn the habits you have adopted in the bid to keep yourself protected-such as avoiding situations that can trigger the attack, which Gideon often did. If the panic attack is beginning to interfere with your normal life, if you have become more timid, or you are avoiding everything that can likely provoke the symptoms, that is the best time to seek professional help.

When panic disorder is at its worst, people with this problem tend to stay at home always to avoid trigger-situations. Sometimes people with panic disorder issues can stop doing what they enjoy doing in an effort to curb the attacks.

Looking Ahead

Gideon maintained that his recovery from panic attack made him a better person and a more helpful person to his friends. While his battle with panic attacks lasted, he was always getting in touch with his friends for help. When he realized he could do well all by himself, he would often call those same friends to share his successes. He said talking to friends about his successes in his battle with panic disorder change the way he talked about his condition. He began to focus more on his recovery rather than his suffering.

Chapter Eight

Overcoming your social anxiety disorder without medications

If you have been dealing with the problem of anxiety disorder, you are not alone as millions of people from different parts of the world have to live with this problem and its attendant symptoms daily. However, you must understand that you don't have to allow the condition deprive you of the fun-filled life you were created to live. One way to overcome social anxiety disorder is to make up your mind to fight the condition with whatever it might cost.

There are several individuals who started life with this problem, but lost it along the line through willful efforts. You might have been born that way, but you don't have to live and die that way. One glaring truth about living with social anxiety disorder is that it will deny of life's most juicy opportunities and events. Living with this problem will keep you in seclusion as you try to avoid the spotlight in order not to be embarrassed.

I have studied the lives of people who live with social anxiety disorder and some others who overcame their social anxiety disorders, and one thing I have come to learn from each one of them is that most times, what they fear do not even exist. Living with social anxiety disorder makes you feel everyone is glaring at you when they are only admiring you. People with social anxiety disorder are quick to judge themselves and come to the conclusion that no one loves them and no one will ever appreciate their efforts.

It is wrong for you to think you are not good enough. The truth is that most of the people you believe are judging you have more serious issues in their lives to deal with and look up to you for some kind of inspiration or motivation. One danger that comes with accepting your social anxiety disorder as your fate for life is that you will never get to know what you are capable of because you never dared to try. All the medications and therapies in the world will not help you get over this problem except you decide to do so.

One way to overcome your social anxiety disorder is to attempt those things you fear the most. Go all out and miss up it won't kill you! Most people with this problem believe they will collapse on stage any day they try to give a public talk or presentation. Social anxiety disorder stops people from achieving anything in life because they believe they will be laughed at for being clumsy. Social anxiety disorder makes you believe you will be too afraid to talk before a crowd, this is called the fear of fear. This is nothing but a state of mind that makes you afraid that you will be frightened the moment you climb on stage and face the crowd.

But the truth remains that things don't always work the way we think when we have these kind of problems. Most people experience stage fright naturally, yet they never fumble the moment they start their presentation. It is all about knowing your limits and daring them. One way to overcome social anxiety disorder is to attempt the very thing you fear most. If what you fear the most is giving a public lecture or presentation, go ahead and do it. Anytime you defy your fears to go on stage, you gain more confidence. The trick is to ignore the hammering of your heart against your rib cage.

People with social anxiety disorder always experience palpitation the moment they face situations they dread the most like giving a public presentation. Someone once told me he thought everyone was listening to the loud thumbing of his heartbeats while he was speaking, but when he ended his presentation, they audience gave him a resounding standing ovation. He was even more amazed when some came up to him to shake his hands for an excellent delivery on stage. Do not think the great orators you listen to never experience stage frights or anxiety before they mount the stage.

It is a natural phenomenon that can be handled efficiently. It becomes a major problem in your life when you start paying more attention to it than you pay to what you are expected to deliver on stage. Preparation is the key. Spend enough time researching on the topic you are to speak of to ensure you know what you are talking about when the time comes. Instead of fear, feel excited about the opportunity to impact knowledge in others. Let this excitement buildup in you and imagine yourself delivering a wonderful piece without mincing words. Practice in front of your mirror while imagining a large crowd before you.

You must have to face a crowd someday so make sure you work on your social anxiety disorder. I know people who missed classes during college days because they feared they might be called to give examples or read out some tests to the class. Such people would never come to class any day they hear there would be a discussion class. They succeeded in dodging situations they were scared of, but they left college with results that could not get them the kind of jobs they desired. Even if you escape giving speeches in school or church, you will still have to give vote of thanks on your wedding day or read a funeral oration at the burial of a parent or loved one.

One way or the other, your fears will still find you out so the best thing to do is to face them. I have listened to great preachers and speakers tell their stories of how they stuttered when they started talking in public gatherings, but listening to them today one would never have imagined they once experienced stage fright. If they could overcome their social anxiety disorders to get to the zenith of their public speaking careers, so can you. Don't say you were born with the problem and there is nothing you can do about it. There are several things you can do about your social anxiety, and the first thing is to decide to become more daring to situations that scare you out of your wits.

Conclusion

One Man's Battle against Social Anxiety Disorder

In my line of work as a life coach and self-improvement expert, I have come across several people with social anxiety disorders. Some of these people were able to overcome their social anxiety disorders after following some of the tips outlined in this book; for some others, nothing they tried was able to help them get rid of social anxiety disorder completely. This affected the latter group of individuals adversely as they were confined to their homes where they felt safe from all kinds of anxiety triggers such as crowded places and public functions.

But one thing I learnt as I observed people suffering social anxiety disorder and how they fought their condition was that nothing is ever lost until you accept that all is lost. One man believed that it was never over until it was over and never got tired of fighting his social anxiety disorder despite the discouraging results his efforts were yielding. Michael was born frail and timid, which was not surprising at all. The frailty was a physical attribute he inherited from his father, while his mother who suffered so much physical, emotional and sexual abuses while a teenager helped groom his timidity as he grew.

Michael grew up believing he was not good enough to compete in life with his peers and age mates. This belief kept him off all kinds of social gatherings an public functions. While in school, Michael had his spot at the back bench where the possibility of any teacher pointing him out for questions and examples were as slim as none. Michael was not the kind of student you could call a dullard, on the contrary, he was a very brilliant student and a fast learner, but his timidity never gave him the confidence to air his views and make his opinions on pressing issues known. Michael was the kind of student that would rather lose some very valuable exam marks than get involved in anything that required him to speak in the class.

At first no one knew what he was battling with until he got admitted into college. In college, he tried to maintain the same life of seclusion he had lived in high school, but it wasn't really working for him because the rules were slightly different. Michael suddenly discovered he couldn't avoid answering some questions and giving some examples during classes. There were classes that required the participation of everyone as a way of keeping record of students' attendance. Michael suddenly saw himself at a crossroad. He could not give up college because so much was at stake, but the confidence required to feature in school activities was one luxury the poor boy could not afford at all.

With time, his teachers noticed he had difficulty remembering anything whenever it was his turn to make presentations or give examples on any given topic. With the help of his psychology professor, he was taken to some therapists and counselor who diagnosed him with social anxiety disorder. The moment he discovered he had a problem, he became resolved to find a lasting solution to his problem, no matter how long it was going to take him and what it would cost.

He started reading books and articles on anxiety disorders and how to handle them.

He bought audio and video tapes from certified professionals, subscribed for daily newsletters on how to deal with the issue, but he was getting little or nothing from all these efforts. The first thought that came to his mind was to throw in the towel as most people do and resort to a life of seclusion and loneliness, but he didn't. He decided to try harder. He changed his therapist and certain behaviors and habits that are believed to be triggers of anxiety.

His new therapist introduced him to several exercises and activities such as deep breathing, meditation, yoga, etc that could help him get the best from his anxiety disorder treatments. His anxiety disorder didn't allow him enjoy all the fun and excitement that can come with college, but he was determined to defy all odds and make the best of his life. Michael understood well the fact that one of the most effective ways to tackle social anxiety disorder is to attempt those very activities that he feared the most. Instead of avoiding dinner nights where he would need to engage some strangers in discussion, he started attending whatever event he got wind of.

Whenever he was in any such event, he tried to engage some other guests in civil discussions. At first it wasn't quite easy for him to strike very interesting conversations, but the more he practiced, the more he mastered the act of talking to others. That experience gave him the confidence to start speaking up in public places such as school gatherings, church events, etc. He got involved in social works that enabled him mix up with more people and make more friends. Before he left college, he was already a master in the act of impressing people and making friends.

On their graduation day, he was one of the best graduating students, and was chosen to make a speech in front of several hundreds of people who had gathered to witness the graduation of their children and wards. Michael prepared well for the speech and gave a very excellent speech that kept the audience transfixed. The audience were mostly learned and well educated men and women from all walks of life who had either come to congratulate some graduating students, witness the event as an alumnus or a friend of the institution. The superb charisma he exuded during the speech won him the heart of several people. That speech marked a new beginning in his life as it helped him discover the orator and public speaker in him.

He was amazed at the number of speaking opportunities that opened to him following that speech. Thus his life as a public speaker and teacher began. His life witnessed an amazing transformation from the very timid and fidgety Michael to a well renowned and reputed public speaker and orator. People say he is one of the best speakers they have ever known due to the way he drives his points home without mincing words. Though he admits that he still feels the fluttering of butterflies in his stomach before he mounts the rostrum in any big event, but it has never stopped him from pursuing his life passion. Today he makes a living just doing what he once feared the most in life-speaking in public. It all goes on to show that where there is a will there will always be a way. If he had given up in high school, he would never know what he was capable of doing on stage. Today, Michael runs a coaching and motivational outfit where he teaches people how to overcome social anxiety disorder and stage frights.

One important lesson to be learnt from Michael's story is that even if you were born with anxiety disorder, you can get rid of it conveniently to live a very normal life doing the things you love to do most. First know the type of anxiety disorder you are dealing with because knowing what you are up against is the first step to defeating it. Once you know which anxiety disorder you are battling with, make sure you talk to your doctor for the best professional advice and treatments. Taking the easy way out, which is avoiding situations that remind you of your past panic attacks is never going to help you become a better you. The best solution to any problem, including your anxiety problems is to take the bull by the horn.

Take the treatments and natural practices your doctor or therapist recommend very serious and make efforts to come out of your shell. Nobody is out to ridicule you and there is no lion or even a wolf after you. The best thing you can do to yourself is to start facing your fears and start doing things you have always feared. Most of the things and situations you are very scared of will never happen because they are not real. Don't forget the importance of maintaining a very healthy mind. You need a positive mindset to get positive results from your treatments and efforts towards becoming more confident and outgoing.

Flush all sorts of dirty and negative thoughts from your mind. Whenever you notice your mind straying towards the negative, find a way to focus on something more positive. Never allow negative thoughts and fears to buildup in your mind. Learn to practice excitement over public events that offer you the chance to mix up and make new friends. Replace your fear of the unknown with excitement. Just convince your mind you are going to have fun in that event, and your mind will start feeding you with positive thoughts. When you refuse to nurture thoughts of fear and why you would not make a good impression, your mind starts believing and acting on it. It will even give you more reasons why you should stay away from that event or situation to save face.

Pay no attention to such negative stream of thoughts. Be brave and defy all fears to conquer your challenges. The best time to start tackling your social anxiety disorder is now because delay is dangerous. I have seen people who contemplated suicide because their anxiety disorders got so bad that they felt they were better off dead than alive. They started believing the lie that their lives would never amount to anything good. This is what happens when you let the social anxiety disorder grow and become severe of the years.

Other books by Publisher and on Audible.com

Hypnotise: The Secret Methods to Hypnosis

The Power of a Curious Mind The Secrets to Master Your Thoughts and Become a Winner!

Breaking The Chains Of A Psycopath And A Sociopath: Learning How to Live Again

Narcissistic Personality Disorder: Narcissistic Men and Women How to Spot Them, Check Them and Then Avoid Them

Charisma: How to Captivate People